I0695494

ACID REFLUX DIET COOKBOOK

SOOTHE GERD AND LPR WITH EASE AND LIVE COMFORTABLY

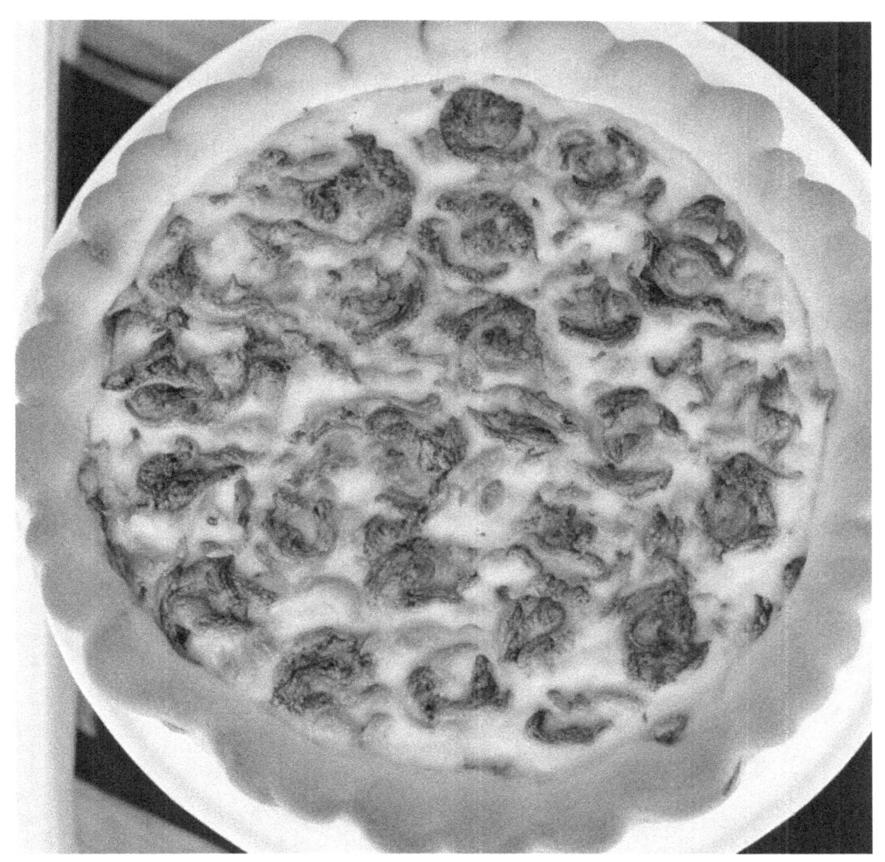

DR CHARLOTTE WASON

All rights reserved. No part of this publication may be reproduced, distributed, or transmitted in any form or by any means, including photocopying, recording, or other electronic or mechanical methods, without the prior written permission of the publisher, except in the case of brief quotations embodied in critical reviews and certain other non-commercial uses permitted by copyright law.

Copyright © 2023 Dr Charlotte Wason

TABLE OF CONTENTS

INTRODUCTION

In a bustling city where the aroma of street food and sizzling delicacies fills the air, there lived a young woman named Emma. She was vivacious, adventurous, and had an insatiable appetite for life's pleasures. But there was one thing that seemed to stand in the way of her boundless spirit - a relentless and unyielding foe known as acid reflux. Like many others, Emma suffered from the discomfort and limitations that came with acid reflux, a condition that had silently woven its way into her daily life. The burning sensation, the taste of acid, and the fear of trigger foods had become her constant companions, dampening her zest for exploration and culinary delights. She yearned for a way to break free from this unwelcome intruder, to embrace life without hesitation, and to reclaim the joy of indulgence she once knew. And so, a journey began - a journey not just to alleviate the symptoms but to find lasting freedom from the clutches of acid reflux. With determination and a desire for change, Emma embarked on a quest to discover the secrets of an acid reflux diet that would not only bring relief but allow her to thrive once again.

In "ACID REFLUX DIET COOKBOOK," we delve into Emma's inspiring story of transformation, set against the backdrop of a mouthwatering culinary adventure. Join us as we explore the hidden gems of a carefully curated acid reflux-friendly diet, packed with delectable recipes and simple lifestyle changes. As her health and happiness begin to soar, Emma finds herself embarking on a new chapter of life - a chapter filled with hope, exploration, and a newfound passion for nourishing her body and soul.

In this comprehensive guide, we unlock the secrets of an acid reflux diet, debunking myths, and equipping you with valuable knowledge to combat this common but often underestimated condition. Each chapter is brimming with delicious recipes, carefully crafted to soothe your digestive system while tantalizing your taste buds. From hearty Mediterranean stews to luscious vegan desserts, we have handpicked the finest recipes that are gentle on your stomach yet rich in flavor. Indulge in the sweet melody of honeyed peaches and the savoriness of lemon herb quinoa, all while knowing you're nurturing your body from within. "Acid Reflux Diet Cookbook" is more than just a cookbook; it's a roadmap to transformation.

Are you ready to embark on your journey to liberation from acid reflux? Let Emma's story inspire you, as we embark on an adventure to discover the art of culinary satisfaction without compromise. The path to freedom awaits within these pages, beckoning you to savor life to the fullest.

Buckle up, dear reader, as we explore the flavors of freedom and indulge in the joy of nourishing our bodies and souls with "ACID REFLUX DIET COOKBOOK." The journey begins now - let the transformation unfold!

CHAPTER 1: WHAT IS ACID REFLUX?

Acid reflux, also known as gastroesophageal reflux disease (GERD), is a condition that occurs when the contents of the stomach flow back into the esophagus. The tube that transports food and liquids from the mouth to the stomach is the esophagus. Normally, a ring of muscle called the lower esophageal sphincter (LES) acts as a valve, opening to allow food and liquids to enter the stomach and closing to prevent stomach contents from flowing back up. In cases of acid reflux, the LES weakens or relaxes inappropriately, allowing stomach acid and sometimes partially digested food to move back into the esophagus. This can lead to irritation and inflammation of the lining of the esophagus, causing symptoms such as heartburn, regurgitation (a bitter or sour taste in the mouth), chest pain, difficulty swallowing, and a chronic cough.

Major Causes Of Acid Reflux

The major causes of acid reflux, also known as gastroesophageal reflux disease (GERD), include:

Hiatal hernia: A hiatal hernia occurs when a part of the stomach pushes up into the chest through the diaphragm. This can weaken the lower esophageal sphincter (LES), the valve that separates the stomach from the esophagus, leading to acid reflux.

Weak lower esophageal sphincter (LES): The LES is a ring of muscle that normally closes to prevent stomach acid from flowing back into the esophagus. If the LES is weak or relaxes inappropriately, it allows stomach acid to reflux into the esophagus.

Dietary factors: Some foods and beverages might contribute to acid reflux. Spicy, fatty, and acidic foods, as well as chocolate, coffee, and carbonated drinks, are common culprits. Tomatoes and citrus fruits can also make symptoms worse.

Overeating: Consuming large meals can put pressure on the stomach and LES, increasing the likelihood of acid reflux.

Lying down after eating: Gravity helps keep stomach contents in the stomach when we stand or sit upright. However, lying down after a meal can make it easier for stomach acid to flow back into the esophagus.

Obesity: Acid reflux might result from the pressure that extra weight can exert on the stomach.

Pregnancy: Hormonal changes during pregnancy and the pressure from a growing uterus can cause acid reflux in pregnant women.

Smoking: Smoking weakens the LES and can increase stomach acid production, contributing to acid reflux.

Certain medications: Some medications, such as antihistamines, calcium channel blockers, and certain asthma medications, can relax the LES or irritate the esophagus, leading to acid reflux.

Alcohol consumption: Excessive alcohol consumption can irritate the esophagus and relax the LES, promoting acid reflux.

Diet And Lifestyle Changes To Reverse Acid Reflux

To help reverse acid reflux and manage gastroesophageal reflux disease (GERD), incorporating the following diet and lifestyle changes can be beneficial:

Avoid Trigger Foods: Identify the foods that cause your acid reflux symptoms and stay away from them. Common triggers include spicy, fatty, and acidic foods, as well as chocolate, coffee, carbonated drinks, citrus fruits, and tomatoes.

Eat Smaller, More Frequent Meals: Consider eating smaller quantities throughout the day rather than large meals. This can reduce pressure on the stomach and LES, minimizing the risk of reflux.

Don't Lie Down After Eating: Avoid lying down immediately after eating. Stay upright for at least 2-3 hours after meals to allow gravity to help keep stomach contents down.

Elevate the Head of Your Bed: Raise the head of your bed by 4-6 inches (10-15 cm) using blocks or a wedge pillow. This can help prevent stomach acid from flowing back into the esophagus while you sleep.

Maintain a Healthy Weight: If you are overweight or obese, losing weight can help reduce pressure on the stomach and improve GERD symptoms.

Quit Smoking: If you smoke, consider quitting. Smoking weakens the LES and increases stomach acid production, contributing to acid reflux.

Limit Alcohol and Caffeine: Reduce alcohol consumption and limit or avoid caffeine-containing beverages as they can exacerbate acid reflux symptoms.

Chew Gum: Chewing sugar-free gum after meals can increase saliva production, which may help neutralize stomach acid and reduce reflux.

Avoid Tight-Fitting Clothing: Tight clothing can exert pressure on the stomach and make acid reflux worse, especially around the waist.

Stay Hydrated: Drink a lot of water all day long. Stomach acid can be diluted with enough hydration.

Wait Before Exercising: Avoid intense exercise or bending over immediately after eating, as these activities can trigger reflux.

Keep a Food Diary: Keeping track of your meals and symptoms in a food diary can help identify specific trigger foods and patterns that worsen your acid reflux.

Consider a GERD-Friendly Diet: Some people find relief by following a GERD-friendly diet, such as a low-acid diet, which includes foods with lower acidity levels.

Manage Stress: Stress can worsen acid reflux symptoms. Exercise deep breathing techniques, yoga, or other stress-relieving hobbies.

Raise the Top of Your Mattress: If elevating the head of your bed is not feasible, you can try placing blocks under the top legs of the bed frame to achieve a slight incline.

When following an acid reflux diet, it's essential to choose foods that are less likely to trigger reflux and avoid those that can worsen symptoms. Here are some guidelines on foods to eat and avoid:

Foods to Eat:

1. Non-acidic Fruits: Opt for fruits with lower acidity levels, such as bananas, melons (watermelon, cantaloupe, honeydew), apples, pears, and mangoes.
2. Non-Citrus Juices: Drink non-citrus juices like apple, pear, or watermelon juice instead of orange, grapefruit, or tomato juice.
3. Vegetables: Most vegetables are well-tolerated, but focus on non-acidic options like leafy greens, broccoli, cauliflower, carrots, and sweet potatoes.
4. Lean Proteins: Choose lean meats like skinless chicken, turkey, fish, and seafood. Eggs and plant-based proteins like tofu can also be good choices.
5. Whole Grains: Opt for whole grains like brown rice, quinoa, oats, and whole wheat bread or pasta.
6. Healthy Fats: Include healthy fats from foods like olive oil, nuts, seeds, and avocados.
7. Low-Fat Dairy: If you tolerate dairy well, choose low-fat options like skim milk, yogurt, or low-fat cheese.
8. Ginger: Ginger can have soothing properties for the digestive system and may help with acid reflux symptoms.
9. Herbal Teas: Non-mint herbal teas like chamomile, licorice, and ginger tea can be soothing and reflux-friendly.
10. Alkaline Water: Some people find relief by drinking alkaline water, which has a higher pH level than regular water.

Foods to Avoid:

1. Acidic Fruits: Citrus fruits like oranges, lemons, grapefruits, and tomatoes can trigger acid reflux.
2. High-Fat Foods: Fatty foods, fried foods, and full-fat dairy products can relax the LES and promote reflux.

3. Spicy Foods: Spices like black pepper, chili powder, and hot sauces may exacerbate symptoms.

4. Mint: Avoid peppermint, spearmint, and mint-flavored foods, as they can relax the LES.

5. Chocolate: Chocolate contains compounds that can worsen reflux symptoms.

6. Carbonated Beverages: Carbonated drinks can contribute to bloating and reflux.

7. Caffeine: Caffeinated beverages like coffee, tea, and sodas can raise stomach acid production.

8. Onions and Garlic: These can be problematic for some individuals with acid reflux.

9. Highly Processed Foods: Processed and fast foods can be high in fat and may contain trigger ingredient

10. Alcohol: Alcoholic beverages can irritate the esophagus and relax the LES.

CHAPTER 2: BREAKFAST RECIPES

Banana Oatmeal

Ingredients:

- 1 ripe banana
- 1/2 cup rolled oats
- 1 cup almond milk (or any non-dairy milk)
- 1 tablespoon honey or maple syrup (optional)
- 1/2 teaspoon ground cinnamon

Procedure:

1. Mash the ripe banana in a saucepan.
2. Add rolled oats and almond milk to the saucepan.
3. Cook over medium heat, stirring occasionally, until the oats are tender and the mixture thickens.
4. Add honey or maple syrup (if using) and ground cinnamon, and stir well.
5. Serve warm.

Veggie Omelette

Ingredients:

- 2 large eggs
- 1/4 cup diced bell peppers (any color)
- 1/4 cup diced tomatoes
- 1/4 cup chopped spinach
- 1 tablespoon olive oil
- Salt and pepper to taste

Procedure:

1. In a bowl, whisk the eggs until well combined.
2. Heat olive oil in a non-stick skillet over medium heat.
3. Add diced bell peppers and sauté for 1-2 minutes.
4. Add diced tomatoes and chopped spinach to the skillet and cook until the vegetables are slightly softened.
5. Pour the whisked eggs over the vegetables in the skillet.
6. Cook until the omelette is set and lightly browned on the bottom.
7. Carefully flip the omelette and cook the other side for a minute.
8. Season with salt and pepper.
9. Serve hot.

Greek Yogurt Parfait

Ingredients:

- 1 cup plain Greek yogurt
- 1/2 cup granola (low-fat and low-sugar)
- 1/2 cup fresh mixed berries (e.g., strawberries, blueberries, raspberries)

Procedure:

1. In a glass or bowl, layer Greek yogurt, granola, and mixed berries.
2. Repeat the layers until all ingredients are used.
3. Finish with a few berries on top for garnish.
4. Serve immediately.

Almond Butter Toast

Ingredients:

- 2 slices whole-grain bread (low-fat)
- 2 tablespoons almond butter
- 1 ripe banana, sliced

Procedure:

1. Toast the slices of whole-grain bread.
2. Spread almond butter evenly on each slice.
3. Top with sliced bananas.
4. Serve as an open-faced sandwich.

Chia Seed Pudding

Ingredients:

- 2 tablespoons chia seeds
- 1 cup almond milk (or any non-dairy milk)
- 1 tablespoon honey or maple syrup (optional)
- 1/2 teaspoon vanilla extract
- Fresh fruit for topping (e.g., berries, sliced kiwi)

Procedure:

1. In a bowl, mix chia seeds, almond milk, honey or maple syrup (if using), and vanilla extract.
2. Stir well to ensure the chia seeds are evenly distributed.
3. Refrigerate the mixture for at least 2 hours or overnight, allowing it to thicken.
4. Before serving, top with fresh fruit.

Apple Cinnamon Smoothie

Ingredients:

- 1 medium apple, peeled and chopped
- 1 cup plain Greek yogurt
- 1/2 cup almond milk (or any non-dairy milk)
- 1/2 teaspoon ground cinnamon
- 1 tablespoon honey or maple syrup (optional)

Procedure:

1. In a blender, combine chopped apple, Greek yogurt, almond milk, ground cinnamon, and honey or maple syrup (if using).
2. Blend until smooth and creamy.
3. Pour into a glass and sprinkle a pinch of cinnamon on top for garnish.
4. Serve immediately.

Quinoa Breakfast Bowl

Ingredients:

- 1/2 cup cooked quinoa
- 1/4 cup sliced almonds
- 1/2 cup mixed berries
- 1 tablespoon honey or maple syrup (optional)

Procedure:

1. In a bowl, combine cooked quinoa, sliced almonds, and mixed berries.
2. Drizzle honey or maple syrup (if using) on top for sweetness.
3. Toss gently to mix all ingredients.

4. Serve at room temperature or slightly warm.

Baked Egg Cups

Ingredients:

- 4 large eggs
- 1 cup baby spinach leaves
- 1/4 cup diced bell peppers (any color)
- Salt and pepper to taste

Procedure:

1. Preheat the oven to 375°F (190°C) and grease a muffin tin.
2. In each muffin cup, place a few baby spinach leaves and diced bell peppers.
3. Crack one egg into each cup, being careful not to break the yolk.
4. Season with salt and pepper.
5. Bake for 12 to 15 minutes, or until the egg whites are set, in the preheated oven.
6. Before removing the egg cups from the muffin container, give them a little time to cool.
7. Serve warm.

Sweet Potato Hash

Ingredients:

- 1 medium sweet potato, peeled and diced
- 1/2 cup diced red onions
- 1/2 cup diced red bell peppers
- 1 tablespoon olive oil
- 1/2 teaspoon paprika
- Salt and pepper to taste

Procedure:

1. In a skillet over medium heat, warm the olive oil.
2. Add diced sweet potato, red onions, and red bell peppers to the skillet.
3. Sprinkle paprika, salt, and pepper over the vegetables.
4. Sauté until the sweet potatoes are tender and slightly caramelized.
5. Serve hot.

Rice Cake with Cottage Cheese and Berries

Ingredients:

- 2 rice cakes (low-sodium)
- 1/2 cup low-fat cottage cheese
- 1/2 cup mixed berries (e.g., strawberries, blueberries, raspberries)

Procedure:

1. Spread a layer of low-fat cottage cheese on each rice cake.
2. Top with mixed berries.
3. Serve as a light and refreshing breakfast option.

CHAPTER 3: LUNCH AND DINNER RECIPES

Baked Salmon with Steamed Vegetables

Ingredients:

- 1 salmon fillet
- 1 tablespoon olive oil
- 1/2 teaspoon dried dill
- 1/2 teaspoon garlic powder
- Salt and pepper to taste
- Assorted steamed vegetables (e.g., broccoli, carrots, zucchini)

Procedure:

1. Preheat the oven to 375°F (190°C).
2. On a baking sheet, put the salmon fillet.
3. Drizzle olive oil over the salmon and sprinkle with dried dill, garlic powder, salt, and pepper.
4. Bake in the preheated oven for about 15-20 minutes or until the salmon is cooked through.
5. Serve with steamed vegetables on the side.

Grilled Chicken Salad

Ingredients:

- 4 ounces grilled chicken breast, sliced
- Mixed salad greens (e.g., spinach, arugula, lettuce)
- 1/4 cup sliced cucumbers
- 1/4 cup cherry tomatoes, halved
- 1/4 avocado, sliced
- Balsamic vinaigrette dressing (low-fat and low-acid)

Procedure:

1. Put the mixed salad greens in a serving dish.
2. Top with sliced grilled chicken, sliced cucumbers, cherry tomatoes, and avocado.
3. Drizzle balsamic vinaigrette dressing over the salad.
4. Toss lightly to combine and serve.

Turkey and Veggie Wrap

Ingredients:

- 2 large whole-grain tortillas (low-fat)
- 4 ounces sliced turkey breast
- 1/4 cup hummus
- 1/4 cup sliced bell peppers (any color)
- 1/4 cup shredded carrots
- 1/4 cup baby spinach leaves

Procedure:

1. On a clean surface, spread the whole-grain tortillas out.
2. Spread hummus evenly on each tortilla.
3. Layer sliced turkey breast, sliced bell peppers, shredded carrots, and baby spinach leaves on top of the hummus.
4. To make wraps, neatly roll the tortillas.
5. Slice the wraps diagonally and serve.

Quinoa Stuffed Bell Peppers

Ingredients:

- 4 large bell peppers (any color)
- 1 cup cooked quinoa
- 1 cup cooked lean ground turkey (seasoned with herbs and spices)
- 1/2 cup diced tomatoes
- 1/4 cup diced red onions
- 1/4 cup shredded low-fat cheese (optional)

Procedure:

1. Preheat the oven to 375°F (190°C).
2. Bell peppers should have the tops cut off and the seeds taken out.
3. In a bowl, mix cooked quinoa, cooked ground turkey, diced tomatoes, and diced red onions.
4. Stuff the mixture into each bell pepper.
5. If using cheese, sprinkle a small amount on top of each stuffed pepper.
6. Place the stuffed peppers in a baking dish.
7. Bake in the preheated oven for about 25-30 minutes or until the peppers are tender.
8. Serve warm.

Lentil and Vegetable Stir-Fry

Ingredients:

- 1 cup cooked lentils
- 1 cup mixed vegetables (e.g., broccoli, bell peppers, snap peas)
- 2 tablespoons low-sodium soy sauce
- 1 tablespoon sesame oil
- 1 clove garlic, minced
- 1 teaspoon grated ginger

- Sesame seeds for garnish

Procedure:

1. Sesame oil should be heated over medium heat in a wok or big skillet.
2. Add grated ginger and minced garlic, stir-fry for a minute until fragrant.
3. Add mixed vegetables to the wok and stir-fry until slightly tender.
4. Stir in cooked lentils and low-sodium soy sauce.
5. Cook for another 2-3 minutes, allowing the flavors to meld.
6. Garnish with sesame seeds and serve.

Baked Cod with Lemon-Herb Sauce

Ingredients:

- 2 cod fillets
- 1 tablespoon olive oil
- 1 lemon, juiced
- 1/2 teaspoon dried thyme
- 1/2 teaspoon dried oregano
- Salt and pepper to taste
- Fresh parsley for garnish

Procedure:

1. Preheat the oven to 375°F (190°C).
2. Cod fillets should be put on a baking sheet.
3. Olive oil and lemon juice should be drizzled over the fillets.
4. Sprinkle dried thyme, dried oregano, salt, and pepper on top.
5. For about 15-20 minutes, or until the cod is cooked through and flakes readily with a fork, bake in the preheated oven.

6. Garnish with fresh parsley and serve.

Eggplant and Zucchini Lasagna

Ingredients:

- 1 large eggplant, thinly sliced
- 2 medium zucchinis, thinly sliced
- 1 cup low-acid tomato sauce (homemade or store-bought)
- 1 cup low-fat ricotta cheese
- 1 cup shredded low-fat mozzarella cheese
- 1/4 cup grated Parmesan cheese
- Fresh basil leaves for garnish

Procedure:

1. Preheat the oven to 375°F (190°C).
2. Spread a thin layer of tomato sauce in the bottom of a baking dish.
3. Layer eggplant slices, zucchini slices, ricotta cheese, and mozzarella cheese in the baking dish.
4. Layers should be repeated until all components have been used.
5. Sprinkle grated Parmesan cheese on top.
6. Cover the dish with foil and bake in the preheated oven for about 30 minutes.
7. Remove the foil and bake for an extra 10 minutes till the cheese is bubbly and golden.
8. Garnish with fresh basil leaves and serve.

Lemon Herb Grilled Chicken

Ingredients:

- 2 boneless, skinless chicken breasts
- 2 tablespoons olive oil
- 1 lemon, juiced and zested
- 1 teaspoon dried rosemary
- 1 teaspoon dried thyme
- Salt and pepper to taste

Procedure:

1. In a bowl, mix olive oil, lemon juice, lemon zest, dried rosemary, dried thyme, salt, and pepper.
2. Add chicken breasts to the bowl and coat them with the marinade.
3. Cover the bowl and refrigerate for at least 30 minutes or up to 4 hours.
4. Grill or grill pan should be preheated at medium heat.
5. Grill the chicken breasts for about 6-7 minutes per side or until cooked through.
6. Prior to serving, let the chicken rest for a few minutes.

Quinoa and Roasted Vegetable Bowl

Ingredients:

- 1 cup cooked quinoa
- Assorted roasted vegetables (e.g., bell peppers, eggplant, cherry tomatoes)
- 2 tablespoons balsamic vinaigrette dressing (low-fat and low-acid)
- 1/4 cup crumbled feta cheese (optional)
- Fresh basil leaves for garnish

Procedure:

1. Cooked quinoa and roasted vegetables should be combined in a bowl.
2. Drizzle balsamic vinaigrette dressing over the quinoa and vegetables.
3. Toss gently to mix all ingredients.
4. Sprinkle the feta cheese, if using, on top.
5. Garnish with fresh basil leaves and serve.

Tofu Stir-Fry with Brown Rice

Ingredients:

- 1 cup cooked brown rice
- 1/2 block firm tofu, cubed
- 1 cup mixed vegetables (e.g., broccoli, bell peppers, snow peas)
- 2 tablespoons low-sodium soy sauce
- 1 tablespoon sesame oil
- 1 clove garlic, minced
- 1 teaspoon grated ginger
- Sesame seeds for garnish

Procedure:

1. Heat sesame oil over medium heat in a wok or big skillet.
2. Add grated ginger and minced garlic then stir-fry for a minute until aromatic.
3. Add mixed vegetables to the wok and stir-fry until slightly tender.
4. Add cubed tofu and low-sodium soy sauce to the wok.
5. Cook for another 2-3 minutes, allowing the flavors to meld.
6. Serve the tofu stir-fry on the cooked brown rice.
7. Garnish with sesame seeds and serve.

CHAPTER 4: MEDITERRANEAN RECIPES

Greek Salad

Ingredients:

- 2 cups mixed salad greens (e.g., lettuce, arugula, spinach)
- 1/2 cucumber, diced
- 1/2 cup cherry tomatoes, halved
- 1/4 cup Kalamata olives, pitted
- 1/4 cup crumbled feta cheese (optional)
- 2 tablespoons extra-virgin olive oil
- 1 tablespoon red wine vinegar
- 1/2 teaspoon dried oregano
- Salt and pepper to taste

Procedure:

1. In a large bowl, combine mixed salad greens, diced cucumber, halved cherry tomatoes, and pitted Kalamata olives.
2. If using feta cheese, add it to the salad.
3. In a separate small bowl, whisk together extra-virgin olive oil, red wine vinegar, dried oregano, salt, and pepper to make the dressing.
4. Drizzle the dressing over the salad and stir to combine.
5. Serve immediately.

Grilled Mediterranean Chicken

Ingredients:

- 2 boneless, skinless chicken breasts
- 2 tablespoons lemon juice
- 2 tablespoons extra-virgin olive oil
- 2 cloves garlic, minced
- 1 teaspoon dried oregano
- 1/2 teaspoon dried thyme
- Salt and pepper to taste

Procedure:

1. In a bowl, mix lemon juice, extra-virgin olive oil, minced garlic, dried oregano, dried thyme, salt, and pepper to make the marinade.
2. Add chicken breasts to the bowl and coat them with the marinade.
3. Cover the bowl and refrigerate for at least 30 minutes or up to 4 hours.
4. Over medium heat, preheat the grill or grill pan.
5. Grill the chicken breasts for about 6-7 minutes per side or until cooked through.
6. Allow the chicken to rest for a few minutes before serving.

Roasted Eggplant and Tomato Pasta

Ingredients:

- 2 cups cooked whole-grain pasta
- 1 medium eggplant, diced
- 1 cup cherry tomatoes, halved
- 2 tablespoons extra-virgin olive oil
- 2 cloves garlic, minced
- 1/2 teaspoon dried basil

- 1/4 teaspoon red pepper flakes (optional)
- Salt and pepper to taste
- Fresh basil leaves for garnish

Procedure:

1. Preheat the oven to 375°F (190°C).
2. In a baking dish, toss diced eggplant and halved cherry tomatoes with extra-virgin olive oil, minced garlic, dried basil, red pepper flakes (if using), salt, and pepper.
3. Roast in the preheated oven for about 20-25 minutes or until the vegetables are tender and slightly caramelized.
4. In a large bowl, combine the roasted eggplant and tomatoes with cooked whole-grain pasta.
5. Garnish with fresh basil leaves and serve.

Lemon Herb Baked Cod

Ingredients:

- 2 cod fillets
- 2 tablespoons extra-virgin olive oil
- 1 lemon, juiced and zested
- 1 teaspoon dried parsley
- 1/2 teaspoon dried thyme
- Salt and pepper to taste

Procedure:

1. Preheat the oven to 375°F (190°C).
2. Cod fillets should be put on a baking pan.
3. Drizzle extra-virgin olive oil and lemon juice over the fillets.
4. Sprinkle dried parsley, dried thyme, salt, and pepper on top.

5. The cod should be baked in the preheated oven for 15 to 20 minutes, or until it is thoroughly cooked and flakes easily with a fork.

6. Garnish with lemon zest and serve.

Mediterranean Quinoa Bowl

Ingredients:

- 1 cup cooked quinoa
- 1/2 cup chickpeas, drained and rinsed
- 1/4 cup diced cucumber
- 1/4 cup cherry tomatoes, halved
- 1/4 cup crumbled feta cheese (optional)
- 2 tablespoons lemon juice
- 2 tablespoons extra-virgin olive oil
- 1 tablespoon chopped fresh parsley
- Salt and pepper to taste

Procedure:

1. In a bowl, combine cooked quinoa, chickpeas, diced cucumber, halved cherry tomatoes, and crumbled feta cheese (if using).

2. In a separate small bowl, whisk together lemon juice, extra-virgin olive oil, chopped fresh parsley, salt, and pepper to make the dressing.

3. Over the quinoa bowl, drizzle the dressing and stir to mix.

4. Serve immediately.

Greek-Style Baked Chicken and Vegetables

Ingredients:

- 2 boneless, skinless chicken breasts
- 1 cup cherry tomatoes, halved
- 1/2 cup pitted Kalamata olives
- 1/4 cup crumbled feta cheese (optional)
- 2 tablespoons extra-virgin olive oil
- 1 tablespoon red wine vinegar
- 1 teaspoon dried oregano
- Salt and pepper to taste

Procedure:

1. Preheat the oven to 375°F (190°C).
2. The chicken breasts should be put on a baking dish.
3. In a bowl, toss halved cherry tomatoes and pitted Kalamata olives with extra-virgin olive oil, red wine vinegar, dried oregano, salt, and pepper.
4. Spread the tomato and olive mixture around the chicken in the baking dish.
5. If using feta cheese, sprinkle it on top of the chicken and vegetables.
6. Bake in the preheated oven for about 25-30 minutes or until the chicken is cooked through.
7. Serve warm.

Shrimp and Zucchini Skewers

Ingredients:

- 1/2 pound large shrimp, peeled and deveined
- 2 small zucchinis, sliced into rounds
- 2 tablespoons extra-virgin olive oil
- 1 tablespoon lemon juice

- 1 teaspoon dried oregano
- Salt and pepper to taste

Procedure:

1. The grill or grill pan should be heated to a medium temperature.
2. In a bowl, mix extra-virgin olive oil, lemon juice, dried oregano, salt, and pepper to make the marinade.
3. Thread the shrimp and zucchini rounds onto skewers.
4. Brush the marinade over the shrimp and zucchini skewers.
5. Grill the skewers for about 2-3 minutes per side or until the shrimp is pink and cooked through.
6. Serve immediately.

Caprese Stuffed Portobello Mushrooms

Ingredients:

- 4 large Portobello mushrooms, stems removed
- 1 cup cherry tomatoes, halved
- 1/2 cup fresh mozzarella balls, halved
- 2 tablespoons extra-virgin olive oil
- 1 tablespoon balsamic vinegar
- 1 tablespoon chopped fresh basil
- Salt and pepper to taste

Procedure:

1. Preheat the oven to 375°F (190°C).
2. In a bowl, mix halved cherry tomatoes and mozzarella balls with extra-virgin olive oil, balsamic vinegar, chopped fresh basil, salt, and pepper.

3. The Portobello mushrooms should be put on a baking pan.

4. Fill each mushroom cap with the tomato and mozzarella mixture.

5. Bake in the preheated oven for about 15-20 minutes or until the mushrooms are tender.

6. Serve warm.

Mediterranean Veggie Pita Pockets

Ingredients:

- 2 whole-grain pita pockets
- 1/2 cup hummus
- 1/2 cup mixed salad greens (e.g., lettuce, arugula, spinach)
- 1/4 cup sliced cucumbers
- 1/4 cup cherry tomatoes, halved
- 1/4 cup sliced red onions
- 1/4 cup crumbled feta cheese (optional)

Procedure:

1. Cut each pita pocket in half to create pockets.
2. Spread hummus inside each pita pocket.
3. Stuff each pocket with mixed salad greens, sliced cucumbers, halved cherry tomatoes, sliced red onions, and crumbled feta cheese (if using).
4. Serve as a refreshing and portable Mediterranean lunch.

Ingredients:

- 1 cup cooked chickpeas, drained and rinsed
- 1/4 cup chopped fresh parsley
- 2 cloves garlic, minced
- 1 teaspoon ground cumin
- 1/2 teaspoon ground coriander
- 1/2 teaspoon baking powder
- Salt and pepper to taste
- 2 tablespoons extra-virgin olive oil

Procedure:

1. Preheat the oven to 375°F (190°C).
2. In a food processor, combine cooked chickpeas, chopped fresh parsley, minced garlic, ground cumin, ground coriander, baking powder, salt, and pepper.
3. The mixture should be thoroughly blended but slightly lumpy after a few pulses.
4. Shape the chickpea mixture into small falafel balls.
5. Place the falafel balls on a baking sheet and drizzle extra-virgin olive oil over them.
6. Bake in the preheated oven for about 20-25 minutes or until the falafel is golden and crispy.
7. Serve the baked falafel with a side of hummus or tahini sauce.

Turkey and Vegetable Stew

Ingredients:

- 1 pound lean ground turkey
- 1 tablespoon olive oil
- 1 cup diced carrots
- 1 cup diced celery
- 1 cup diced zucchini
- 1 cup diced bell peppers (any color)
- 2 cloves garlic, minced
- 4 cups low-sodium chicken broth
- 1 teaspoon dried thyme
- Salt and pepper to taste

Procedure:

1. Olive oil is heated over medium heat in a big pot.
2. For one minute, sauté the minced garlic until aromatic.\
3. Add ground turkey to the pot and cook until browned, breaking it apart with a spoon.
4. Stir in diced carrots, celery, zucchini, and bell peppers.
5. Pour low-sodium chicken broth into the pot and add dried thyme, salt, and pepper.
6. Bring the stew to a simmer and let it cook for about 20-25 minutes until the vegetables are tender.
7. Serve the turkey and vegetable stew hot.

Lentil and Spinach Stew

Ingredients:

- 1 cup dried lentils, rinsed and drained
- 1 tablespoon olive oil
- 1 cup chopped onions
- 2 cloves garlic, minced
- 4 cups low-sodium vegetable broth
- 1 teaspoon ground cumin
- 1/2 teaspoon ground coriander
- 2 cups chopped fresh spinach
- Salt and pepper to taste

Procedure:

1. Olive oil is heated in a sizable pot over a medium flame.
2. Add chopped onions and sauté until translucent.
3. Add the minced garlic and stir until fragrant, about one more minute.
4. Add dried lentils to the pot and pour in low-sodium vegetable broth.
5. Add salt, pepper, ground cumin, and ground coriander to season.
6. The stew should be heated to a boil, then simmer for 20 to 25 minutes, or until the lentils are soft.
7. Add chopped fresh spinach to the stew and cook for a few more minutes until wilted.
8. Serve the lentil and spinach stew hot.

Ingredients:

- 1 pound boneless, skinless chicken thighs, cut into chunks
- 1 tablespoon olive oil
- 1 cup sliced mushrooms
- 1 cup diced onions
- 2 cloves garlic, minced
- 4 cups low-sodium chicken broth
- 1 teaspoon dried thyme
- 1/2 teaspoon dried rosemary
- Salt and pepper to taste

Procedure:

1. Olive oil is heated in a big saucepan at a medium temperature.
2. Add diced onions and sauté until softened.
3. Stir in minced garlic and sliced mushrooms, and cook until the mushrooms are tender.
4. Add the chicken chunks to the pot and cook until browned on all sides.
5. Pour low-sodium chicken broth into the pot and season with dried thyme, dried rosemary, salt, and pepper.
6. Bring the stew to a simmer and let it cook for about 20-25 minutes or until the chicken is cooked through and tender.
7. Serve the chicken and mushroom stew hot.

Tomato Basil Sauce

Ingredients:

- 2 cups diced tomatoes (fresh or canned)
- 2 cloves garlic, minced
- 2 tablespoons olive oil
- 1/4 cup chopped fresh basil leaves
- 1/2 teaspoon dried oregano
- Salt and pepper to taste

Procedure:

1. Olive oil should be heated in a pan over medium heat.
2. Sauté the minced garlic for one minute or until fragrant.
3. Stir in diced tomatoes and dried oregano, and let the sauce simmer for about 10-15 minutes until the tomatoes break down and thicken.
4. Add chopped fresh basil to the sauce and season with salt and pepper.
5. Continue simmering for a few more minutes until the flavors meld.
6. Serve the tomato basil sauce over cooked pasta, chicken, or fish.

Lemon Dill Sauce

Ingredients:

- 1/2 cup plain Greek yogurt
- 1 tablespoon lemon juice
- 1 teaspoon dried dill
- 1 clove garlic, minced
- Salt and pepper to taste

Procedure:

1. In a bowl, mix plain Greek yogurt, lemon juice, dried dill, minced garlic, salt, and pepper.
2. Stir well until all ingredients are combined.
3. Serve the lemon dill sauce as a topping for grilled chicken, fish, or vegetables.

Roasted Red Pepper Sauce

Ingredients:

- 2 large red bell peppers, roasted and peeled
- 2 cloves garlic, minced
- 2 tablespoons olive oil
- 1/4 cup low-sodium vegetable broth
- 1/4 cup chopped fresh parsley
- Salt and pepper to taste

Procedure:

1. In a blender or food processor, combine roasted red bell peppers, minced garlic, olive oil, and low-sodium vegetable broth.
2. Blend until smooth and creamy.
3. Stir in chopped fresh parsley and season with salt and pepper.
4. Serve the roasted red pepper sauce over grilled chicken, fish, or pasta.

Creamy Cauliflower Sauce

Ingredients:

- 2 cups cooked cauliflower florets
- 1 cup low-sodium chicken broth (or vegetable broth)
- 2 cloves garlic, minced
- 2 tablespoons olive oil
- 1/4 cup grated Parmesan cheese
- Salt and pepper to taste

Procedure:

1. In a blender or food processor, combine cooked cauliflower florets, minced garlic, olive oil, and low-sodium chicken broth.
2. Blend until smooth and creamy.
3. Season with salt and pepper and stir in the grated Parmesan cheese.
4. Serve the creamy cauliflower sauce over cooked pasta, chicken, or vegetables.

Cilantro Lime Sauce

Ingredients:

- 1 cup fresh cilantro leaves
- 1/4 cup plain Greek yogurt
- 2 tablespoons lime juice
- 1 clove garlic, minced
- 1/2 teaspoon ground cumin
- Salt and pepper to taste

Procedure:

1. In a blender or food processor, combine fresh cilantro leaves, plain Greek yogurt, lime juice, minced garlic, ground cumin, salt, and pepper.
2. Blend until smooth and creamy.
3. Serve the cilantro lime sauce as a topping for grilled chicken, fish, or tacos.

Chunky Vegetable Stew

Ingredients:

- 1 tablespoon olive oil
- 1 cup diced onions
- 1 cup diced carrots
- 1 cup diced celery
- 1 cup diced zucchini
- 1 cup diced bell peppers (any color)
- 2 cloves garlic, minced
- 4 cups low-sodium vegetable broth
- 1 teaspoon dried thyme
- 1/2 teaspoon dried rosemary
- Salt and pepper to taste

Procedure:

1. Olive oil should be heated over medium heat in a big pot.
2. Add diced onions and sauté until softened.
3. Olive oil should be heated in a sizable pot over a medium flame.
4. Pour low-sodium vegetable broth into the pot and season with dried thyme, dried rosemary, salt, and pepper.
5. Bring the stew to a simmer and let it cook for about 20-25 minutes or until the vegetables are tender.

6. Serve the chunky vegetable stew hot.

White Bean and Tomato Stew

Ingredients:

- 2 tablespoons olive oil
- 1 cup diced onions
- 2 cloves garlic, minced
- 1 can (15 ounces) white beans, drained and rinsed
- 1 can (15 ounces) diced tomatoes (low-acid or no-salt-added)
- 2 cups low-sodium vegetable broth
- 1 teaspoon dried thyme
- 1/2 teaspoon dried rosemary
- Salt and pepper to taste

Procedure:

1. Olive oil should be heated in a sizable pot over a medium flame.
2. Add diced onions and sauté until softened.
3. Add the minced garlic and stir until fragrant, about one more minute.
4. Add white beans and diced tomatoes to the pot.
5. Pour low-sodium vegetable broth into the pot and season with dried thyme, dried rosemary, salt, and pepper.
6. Bring the stew to a simmer and let it cook for about 15-20 minutes to allow the flavors to meld.
7. Serve the white bean and tomato stew hot.

CHAPTER 6: WHOLE GRAIN RECIPES

Quinoa and Vegetable Stir-Fry

Ingredients:

- 1 cup cooked quinoa
- 1 cup mixed vegetables (e.g., broccoli, bell peppers, snap peas)
- 2 tablespoons low-sodium soy sauce
- 1 tablespoon sesame oil
- 1 clove garlic, minced
- 1 teaspoon grated ginger
- Sesame seeds for garnish

Procedure:

1. Sesame oil should be heated over medium heat in a wok or big skillet.
2. Grated ginger and minced garlic should be stir-fried for one minute, or until aromatic.
3. Add mixed vegetables to the wok and stir-fry until slightly tender.
4. Add the low-sodium soy sauce and cooked quinoa.
5. Cook for another 2-3 minutes, allowing the flavors to meld.
6. Garnish with sesame seeds and serve.

Brown Rice and Lentil Salad

Ingredients:

- 1 cup cooked brown rice
- 1 cup cooked lentils
- 1/4 cup chopped cucumber
- 1/4 cup diced red bell pepper
- 1/4 cup chopped fresh parsley

- 2 tablespoons extra-virgin olive oil
- 1 tablespoon lemon juice
- Salt and pepper to taste

Procedure:

1. In a large bowl, combine cooked brown rice, cooked lentils, chopped cucumber, diced red bell pepper, and chopped fresh parsley.
2. In a separate small bowl, whisk together extra-virgin olive oil, lemon juice, salt, and pepper to make the dressing.
3. Drizzle the dressing over the rice and lentil mixture.
4. Toss to combine and serve the salad.

Whole Wheat Pasta with Roasted Vegetables

Ingredients:

- 2 cups cooked whole wheat pasta
- 1 cup chopped zucchini
- 1 cup chopped eggplant
- 1 cup cherry tomatoes, halved
- 2 tablespoons extra-virgin olive oil
- 2 cloves garlic, minced
- 1/2 teaspoon dried oregano
- Salt and pepper to taste

Procedure:

1. Preheat the oven to 375°F (190°C).
2. In a baking dish, toss chopped zucchini, eggplant, and halved cherry tomatoes with extra-virgin olive oil, minced garlic, dried oregano, salt, and pepper.

3. Roast in the preheated oven for about 20-25 minutes or until the vegetables are tender and slightly caramelized.

4. In a large bowl, combine the roasted vegetables with cooked whole wheat pasta.

5. Serve the pasta with roasted vegetables warm.

Quinoa and Black Bean Tacos

Ingredients:

- 1 cup cooked quinoa
- 1 cup cooked black beans, drained and rinsed
- 1/2 cup diced tomatoes
- 1/4 cup diced red onions
- 1/4 cup chopped fresh cilantro
- 1 tablespoon lime juice
- 1 teaspoon ground cumin
- Salt and pepper to taste
- Whole grain taco shells or tortillas

Procedure:

1. In a bowl, mix cooked quinoa, cooked black beans, diced tomatoes, diced red onions, chopped fresh cilantro, lime juice, ground cumin, salt, and pepper.

2. Warm the whole grain taco shells or tortillas according to package instructions.

3. Fill each taco shell with the quinoa and black bean mixture.

4. Serve the quinoa and black bean tacos with additional toppings such as avocado slices, lettuce, or salsa if desired.

Ingredients:

- 1 cup cooked bulgur
- 1 cup cooked chickpeas, drained and rinsed
- 1/4 cup chopped fresh mint leaves
- 1/4 cup chopped fresh parsley
- 1/4 cup chopped red onions
- 2 tablespoons extra-virgin olive oil
- 1 tablespoon lemon juice
- Salt and pepper to taste

Procedure:

1. In a large bowl, combine cooked bulgur, cooked chickpeas, chopped fresh mint, chopped fresh parsley, and chopped red onions.
2. In a separate small bowl, whisk together extra-virgin olive oil, lemon juice, salt, and pepper to make the dressing.
3. Drizzle the dressing over the bulgur and chickpea mixture.
4. Toss to combine and serve the bulgur salad.

Ingredients:

- 1 cup cooked farro
- 1 cup chopped roasted vegetables (e.g., sweet potatoes, Brussels sprouts, red onions)
- 2 tablespoons balsamic vinaigrette dressing (low-fat and low-acid)
- 1/4 cup crumbled feta cheese (optional)
- Fresh basil leaves for garnish

Procedure:

1. In a bowl, combine cooked farro and chopped roasted vegetables.
2. Drizzle balsamic vinaigrette dressing over the farro and vegetables.
3. Sprinkle the feta cheese on top if you're using it.
4. Garnish with fresh basil leaves and serve.

Ingredients:

- 1 cup cooked barley
- 4 cups low-sodium vegetable broth
- 1 cup chopped mixed vegetables (e.g., carrots, celery, green beans)
- 1 cup chopped tomatoes (low-acid or no-salt-added)
- 1/2 teaspoon dried thyme
- Salt and pepper to taste

Procedure:

1. In a large pot, bring low-sodium vegetable broth to a boil.
2. Add chopped mixed vegetables and chopped tomatoes to the pot.

3. Stir in cooked barley and dried thyme.

4. Season with salt and pepper to taste.

5. Simmer the soup for about 15-20 minutes until the vegetables are tender and the flavors meld.

6. Serve the barley and vegetable soup hot.

Brown Rice and Vegetable Sushi Rolls

Ingredients:

- 4 nori seaweed sheets
- 2 cups cooked brown rice
- 1/2 cup sliced cucumber
- 1/2 avocado, sliced
- 1/4 cup shredded carrots
- 1/4 cup sliced bell peppers (any color)
- Pickled ginger, wasabi, and low-sodium soy sauce for serving (optional)

Procedure:

1. Lay out a bamboo sushi rolling mat and place a nori seaweed sheet on top.

2. Spread a thin layer of cooked brown rice over the nori sheet, leaving about an inch of space at the top.

3. Arrange sliced cucumber, avocado, shredded carrots, and sliced bell peppers in a line across the rice.

4. Carefully roll up the sushi using the bamboo mat, pressing gently to shape it.

5. Wet the top edge of the nori sheet with water to seal the sushi roll.

6. To produce more sushi rolls, repeat the process.

7. Slice the sushi rolls into bite-sized pieces using a sharp knife.

8. Serve the brown rice and vegetable sushi rolls with pickled ginger, wasabi, and low-sodium soy sauce if desired.

Buckwheat Noodles with Sesame Sauce

Ingredients:

- 2 cups cooked buckwheat noodles (soba noodles)
- 2 tablespoons sesame oil
- 2 tablespoons low-sodium soy sauce
- 1 tablespoon rice vinegar
- 1 tablespoon honey or maple syrup
- 1 tablespoon toasted sesame seeds
- Sliced green onions and shredded carrots for garnish

Procedure:

1. In a bowl, whisk together sesame oil, low-sodium soy sauce, rice vinegar, honey or maple syrup, and toasted sesame seeds to make the sauce.
2. Cook buckwheat noodles according to package instructions and drain.
3. Toss the cooked noodles with the sesame sauce until well coated.
4. Garnish with sliced green onions and shredded carrots.
5. Serve the buckwheat noodles with sesame sauce warm or cold.

Quinoa Stuffed Bell Peppers

Ingredients:

- 4 bell peppers (any color), tops removed and seeds removed
- 1 cup cooked quinoa
- 1 cup diced tomatoes (low-acid or no-salt-added)
- 1 cup cooked black beans, drained and rinsed
- 1/4 cup chopped fresh cilantro
- 1 teaspoon ground cumin

- Salt and pepper to taste
- Olive oil for drizzling

Procedure:

1. Preheat the oven to 375°F (190°C).
2. In a bowl, mix cooked quinoa, diced tomatoes, cooked black beans, chopped fresh cilantro, ground cumin, salt, and pepper.
3. Stuff the quinoa mixture inside each bell pepper.
4. Drizzle a little olive oil over the stuffed bell peppers.
5. Place the stuffed bell peppers in a baking dish and bake in the preheated oven for about 25-30 minutes or until the peppers are tender.
6. Serve the quinoa stuffed bell peppers hot.

CHAPTER 7: VEGAN AND VEGETARIAN RECIPES

Chickpea and Vegetable Curry

Ingredients:

- 1 can (15 ounces) chickpeas, drained and rinsed
- 1 cup diced tomatoes (low-acid or no-salt-added)
- 1 cup diced carrots
- 1 cup diced bell peppers (any color)
- 1 cup diced zucchini
- 1 cup diced onions
- 2 cloves garlic, minced
- 1 can (13.5 ounces) coconut milk
- 2 tablespoons curry powder
- 1 tablespoon olive oil
- Salt and pepper to taste
- Fresh cilantro for garnish

Procedure:

1. Olive oil is heated over medium heat in a big pot.
2. Add the minced garlic and cook it for a minute, until it becomes aromatic.
3. Stir in diced onions and cook until softened.
4. Add diced carrots, bell peppers, and zucchini to the pot, and cook until slightly tender.
5. Pour in diced tomatoes, chickpeas, coconut milk, and curry powder.
6. Season with salt and pepper to taste.
7. Simmer the curry for about 15-20 minutes until the vegetables are cooked through and the flavors meld.
8. Garnish with fresh cilantro and serve the chickpea and vegetable curry over cooked brown rice or quinoa.

Lentil Shepherd's Pie

Ingredients:

- 1 cup cooked lentils
- 1 cup diced carrots
- 1 cup diced celery
- 1 cup diced onions
- 2 cloves garlic, minced
- 1 cup vegetable broth
- 2 tablespoons tomato paste (low-acid)
- 1 tablespoon olive oil
- 2 cups mashed sweet potatoes (cooked and mashed without butter or cream)
- Salt and pepper to taste

Procedure:

1. In a large skillet set over medium heat, olive oil should be heated.
2. Add the minced garlic and cook it for a minute, until it becomes aromatic.
3. Stir in diced onions and cook until softened.
4. Add diced carrots and celery to the skillet, and cook until slightly tender.
5. Pour in vegetable broth, cooked lentils, and tomato paste.
6. Season with salt and pepper to taste.
7. Simmer the mixture for about 10-15 minutes until the vegetables are cooked through and the flavors meld.
8. Preheat the oven to 375°F (190°C).
9. In a baking dish, spread the lentil and vegetable mixture evenly.
10. Top the mixture with mashed sweet potatoes.
11. Bake in the preheated oven for about 15-20 minutes or until the sweet potato topping is lightly browned.
12. Serve the lentil shepherd's pie hot.

Vegan Cauliflower Alfredo Pasta

Ingredients:

- 2 cups cooked whole grain pasta
- 2 cups cauliflower florets, cooked and softened
- 1 cup unsweetened almond milk
- 2 tablespoons nutritional yeast
- 1 tablespoon olive oil
- 2 cloves garlic, minced
- 1/2 teaspoon dried thyme
- Salt and pepper to taste

Procedure:

1. In a blender or food processor, combine cooked cauliflower florets, unsweetened almond milk, nutritional yeast, minced garlic, olive oil, dried thyme, salt, and pepper.
2. Blend until smooth and creamy, adding more almond milk if needed to reach the desired consistency.
3. In a separate pot, warm the cauliflower Alfredo sauce over low heat.
4. Add cooked whole grain pasta to the pot and toss to coat the pasta with the sauce.
5. Serve the vegan cauliflower Alfredo pasta with a sprinkle of additional nutritional yeast and fresh parsley if desired.

Stuffed Bell Peppers with Quinoa and Black Beans

Ingredients:

- 4 bell peppers (any color), tops removed and seeds removed
- 1 cup cooked quinoa
- 1 cup cooked black beans, drained and rinsed
- 1 cup diced tomatoes (low-acid or no-salt-added)
- 1/2 cup diced onions
- 2 cloves garlic, minced
- 1 teaspoon ground cumin
- Salt and pepper to taste
- Olive oil for drizzling

Procedure:

1. Preheat the oven to 375°F (190°C).
2. In a bowl, mix cooked quinoa, cooked black beans, diced tomatoes, diced onions, minced garlic, ground cumin, salt, and pepper.
3. Fill the quinoa and black bean mixture inside of each bell pepper.
4. Drizzle a little olive oil over the stuffed bell peppers.
5. Place the stuffed bell peppers in a baking dish and bake in the preheated oven for about 25-30 minutes or until the peppers are tender.
6. Serve the stuffed bell peppers hot.

Vegan Lentil Bolognese

Ingredients:

- 1 cup cooked lentils
- 1 cup diced carrots
- 1 cup diced celery
- 1 cup diced onions
- 2 cloves garlic, minced
- 1 can (15 ounces) crushed tomatoes (low-acid or no-salt-added)
- 2 tablespoons tomato paste (low-acid)
- 2 tablespoons olive oil
- 1 teaspoon dried oregano
- 1/2 teaspoon dried basil
- Salt and pepper to taste
- Whole grain spaghetti or pasta of your choice

Procedure:

1. In a large skillet set over medium heat, olive oil should be heated.
2. Add the minced garlic and cook it for a minute, until it becomes aromatic.
3. Stir in diced onions and cook until softened.
4. Add diced carrots and celery to the skillet, and cook until slightly tender.
5. Pour in crushed tomatoes, cooked lentils, and tomato paste.
6. Add salt, pepper, dried basil, and dry oregano to season.
7. Simmer the lentil Bolognese sauce for about 15-20 minutes until the flavors meld.
8. Cook whole grain spaghetti or pasta according to package instructions and drain.
9. The cooked pasta should be served and topped with the vegan lentil Bolognese sauce.

Quinoa and Black Bean Salad

Ingredients:

- 1 cup cooked quinoa
- 1 cup cooked black beans, drained and rinsed
- 1/2 cup diced red bell pepper
- 1/4 cup diced red onions
- 1/4 cup chopped fresh cilantro
- 2 tablespoons lime juice
- 2 tablespoons olive oil
- Salt and pepper to taste

Procedure:

1. In a large bowl, combine cooked quinoa, cooked black beans, diced red bell pepper, diced red onions, and chopped fresh cilantro.
2. To create the dressing, combine the lime juice, olive oil, salt, and pepper in a separate small bowl.
3. Drizzle the dressing over the quinoa and black bean salad.
4. Toss to combine and serve the salad.

Vegan Lentil Chili

Ingredients:

- 1 cup cooked lentils
- 1 cup diced tomatoes (low-acid or no-salt-added)
- 1 cup diced bell peppers (any color)
- 1 cup diced zucchini
- 1 cup diced onions
- 2 cloves garlic, minced

- 1 can (15 ounces) kidney beans, drained and rinsed

- 1 can (15 ounces) black beans, drained and rinsed

- 4 cups low-sodium vegetable broth

- 2 tablespoons chili powder

- 1 teaspoon ground cumin

- Salt and pepper to taste

Procedure:

1. Olive oil is heated in a sizable pot over a medium temperature.
2. Add the minced garlic and cook it for a minute, until it becomes aromatic.
3. Stir in diced onions and cook until softened.
4. Add diced bell peppers and zucchini to the pot, and cook until slightly tender.
5. Pour in diced tomatoes, cooked lentils, kidney beans, black beans, low-sodium vegetable broth, chili powder, ground cumin, salt, and pepper.
6. Bring the chili to a simmer and let it cook for about 20-25 minutes until the flavors meld.
7. Serve the vegan lentil chili hot.

Spinach and Mushroom Quiche

Ingredients:

- 1 whole wheat pie crust (store-bought or homemade)

- 2 cups fresh spinach leaves

- 1 cup sliced mushrooms

- 1 cup diced onions

- 2 cloves garlic, minced

- 1 cup unsweetened almond milk

- 1/4 cup nutritional yeast

- 1 tablespoon olive oil

- 1/2 teaspoon dried thyme

- Salt and pepper to taste

Procedure:

1. Preheat the oven to 375°F (190°C).
2. In a skillet set over medium heat, olive oil should be heated.
3. Add the minced garlic and cook it for a minute, until it becomes aromatic.
4. Stir in diced onions and cook until softened.
5. Add sliced mushrooms and fresh spinach leaves to the skillet, and cook until the vegetables are wilted.
6. In a separate bowl, whisk together unsweetened almond milk, nutritional yeast, dried thyme, salt, and pepper to make the quiche filling.
7. In the whole wheat pie crust, spread the sautéed vegetables evenly.
8. Pour the quiche filling over the vegetables.
9. Bake the quiche in the preheated oven for 30-35 minutes, or until it has set and the top is just beginning to brown.
10. Serve the spinach and mushroom quiche warm.

Vegan Sweet Potato and Black Bean Quesadillas

Ingredients:

- 4 whole grain tortillas
- 1 cup mashed sweet potatoes (cooked and mashed without butter or cream)
- 1 cup cooked black beans, drained and rinsed
- 1/2 cup diced tomatoes (low-acid or no-salt-added)
- 1/4 cup diced red onions
- 1/4 cup chopped fresh cilantro
- 1 tablespoon olive oil
- Salt and pepper to taste
- Guacamole and salsa for serving (optional)

Procedure:

1. In a bowl, mix mashed sweet potatoes, cooked black beans, diced tomatoes, diced red onions, chopped fresh cilantro, olive oil, salt, and pepper.
2. Lay out a whole grain tortilla and spread a layer of the sweet potato and black bean mixture on one half.
3. To make a quesadilla, fold the second half of the tortilla over the filling.
4. Repeat the process to make more quesadillas.
5. Olive oil is heated in a skillet at a medium temperature.
6. Cook each quesadilla for a few minutes on each side until lightly browned and crispy.
7. Serve the vegan sweet potato and black bean quesadillas with guacamole and salsa if desired.

Vegan Stuffed Portobello Mushrooms

Ingredients:

- 4 large Portobello mushrooms, stems removed
- 1 cup cooked quinoa
- 1 cup diced tomatoes (low-acid or no-salt-added)
- 1 cup chopped spinach
- 1/2 cup diced red onions
- 2 cloves garlic, minced
- 2 tablespoons balsamic vinegar (low-acid)
- 2 tablespoons olive oil
- Salt and pepper to taste
- Vegan cheese shreds for topping (optional)

Procedure:

1. Preheat the oven to 375°F (190°C).
2. In a large bowl, combine cooked quinoa, diced tomatoes, chopped spinach, diced red onions, minced garlic, balsamic vinegar, olive oil, salt, and pepper.

3. The Portobello mushrooms should be put on a baking pan.

4. The mixture of quinoa and vegetables should be put inside each mushroom cap.

5. If desired, sprinkle vegan cheese shreds on top of each stuffed mushroom.

6. Bake in the preheated oven for about 15-20 minutes or until the mushrooms are tender.

7. Serve the vegan stuffed Portobello mushrooms hot.

Cucumber and Avocado Salad

Ingredients:

- 1 large cucumber, thinly sliced
- 1 ripe avocado, diced
- 1/4 cup diced red onions
- 2 tablespoons chopped fresh dill
- 2 tablespoons olive oil
- 1 tablespoon lemon juice
- Salt and pepper to taste

Procedure:

1. In a large bowl, combine thinly sliced cucumber, diced avocado, diced red onions, and chopped fresh dill.
2. In a separate small bowl, whisk together olive oil, lemon juice, salt, and pepper to make the dressing.
3. Drizzle the dressing over the cucumber and avocado mixture.
4. Toss to combine and serve the cucumber and avocado salad.

Roasted Vegetable Medley

Ingredients:

- 2 cups mixed vegetables (e.g., bell peppers, zucchini, cherry tomatoes)
- 1 tablespoon olive oil
- 1/2 teaspoon dried oregano
- 1/2 teaspoon dried thyme
- Salt and pepper to taste

Procedure:

1. Preheat the oven to 400°F (200°C).
2. In a baking dish, toss mixed vegetables with olive oil, dried oregano, dried thyme, salt, and pepper.
3. The veggies should be roasted in the preheated oven for 15 to 20 minutes, or until they are soft and just beginning to caramelize.
4. The roasted vegetable medley should be served as a side dish.

Quinoa and Pomegranate Salad

Ingredients:

- 1 cup cooked quinoa
- 1/2 cup pomegranate arils
- 1/4 cup chopped fresh mint leaves
- 1/4 cup chopped fresh parsley
- 2 tablespoons olive oil
- 1 tablespoon lemon juice
- Salt and pepper to taste

Procedure:

1. In a large bowl, combine cooked quinoa, pomegranate arils, chopped fresh mint, and chopped fresh parsley.
2. In a separate small bowl, whisk together olive oil, lemon juice, salt, and pepper to make the dressing.
3. Drizzle the dressing over the quinoa and pomegranate mixture.
4. Toss to combine and serve the quinoa and pomegranate salad.

Balsamic Roasted Brussels Sprouts

Ingredients:

- 2 cups Brussels sprouts, trimmed and halved
- 2 tablespoons balsamic vinegar (low-acid)
- 1 tablespoon olive oil
- 1/2 teaspoon dried thyme
- Salt and pepper to taste

Procedure:

1. Preheat the oven to 400°F (200°C).
2. In a baking dish, toss halved Brussels sprouts with balsamic vinegar, olive oil, dried thyme, salt, and pepper.
3. Roast in the preheated oven for about 15-20 minutes or until the Brussels sprouts are tender and slightly caramelized.
4. Serve the balsamic roasted Brussels sprouts as a side dish.

Spinach and Strawberry Salad

Ingredients:

- 2 cups fresh spinach leaves
- 1 cup sliced strawberries
- 1/4 cup sliced almonds
- 2 tablespoons balsamic vinaigrette dressing (low-acid)
- Salt and pepper to taste

Procedure:

1. In a large bowl, combine fresh spinach leaves, sliced strawberries, and sliced almonds.
2. Drizzle balsamic vinaigrette dressing over the salad.
3. Toss to combine and serve the spinach and strawberry salad.

Lemon Herb Quinoa

Ingredients:

- 1 cup cooked quinoa
- 1 tablespoon olive oil
- 2 tablespoons lemon juice
- 1 tablespoon chopped fresh parsley
- 1 tablespoon chopped fresh mint leaves
- Salt and pepper to taste

Procedure:

1. In a bowl, mix cooked quinoa with olive oil, lemon juice, chopped fresh parsley, chopped fresh mint, salt, and pepper.
2. Serve the lemon herb quinoa as a side dish.

Tomato and Cucumber Salad

Ingredients:

- 1 cup diced tomatoes (low-acid or no-salt-added)
- 1 cup diced cucumbers
- 1/4 cup diced red onions
- 2 tablespoons chopped fresh basil
- 2 tablespoons olive oil

- 1 tablespoon red wine vinegar (low-acid)

- Salt and pepper to taste

Procedure:

1. In a large bowl, combine diced tomatoes, diced cucumbers, diced red onions, and chopped fresh basil.

2. In a separate small bowl, whisk together olive oil, red wine vinegar, salt, and pepper to make the dressing.

3. Drizzle the dressing over the tomato and cucumber mixture.

4. Toss to combine and serve the tomato and cucumber salad.

CHAPTER 9: SEAFOOD RECIPES

Baked Lemon Herb Salmon

Ingredients:

- 2 salmon fillets
- 2 tablespoons olive oil
- 2 tablespoons lemon juice
- 1 tablespoon chopped fresh dill
- 1 tablespoon chopped fresh parsley
- 1 clove garlic, minced
- Salt and pepper to taste
- Lemon slices for garnish

Procedure:

1. Preheat the oven to 375°F (190°C).
2. In a small bowl, whisk together olive oil, lemon juice, chopped fresh dill, chopped fresh parsley, minced garlic, salt, and pepper.
3. Place the salmon fillets in a baking dish and drizzle the lemon herb mixture over them.
4. Bake in the preheated oven for about 15-20 minutes or until the salmon is cooked through.
5. Garnish with lemon slices and serve the baked lemon herb salmon.

Grilled Shrimp Skewers

Ingredients:

- 1 pound large shrimp, peeled and deveined
- 2 tablespoons olive oil
- 1 tablespoon lemon juice
- 1 teaspoon paprika

- 1/2 teaspoon garlic powder

- 1/2 teaspoon dried oregano

- Salt and pepper to taste

Procedure:

1. In a bowl, toss the peeled and deveined shrimp with olive oil, lemon juice, paprika, garlic powder, dried oregano, salt, and pepper.
2. Thread the seasoned shrimp onto skewers.
3. Grill or grill pan should be preheated at medium-high heat.
4. Grill the shrimp skewers for about 2-3 minutes on each side or until they are opaque and cooked through.
5. Serve the grilled shrimp skewers hot.

Tuna and White Bean Salad

Ingredients:

- 1 can (5 ounces) tuna, drained

- 1 can (15 ounces) white beans, drained and rinsed

- 1/4 cup diced red onions

- 2 tablespoons chopped fresh parsley

- 2 tablespoons lemon juice

- 1 tablespoon olive oil

- Salt and pepper to taste

Procedure:

1. In a bowl, mix the drained tuna, white beans, diced red onions, chopped fresh parsley, lemon juice, olive oil, salt, and pepper.
2. Toss to combine and serve the tuna and white bean salad.

Baked Cod with Herbs

Ingredients:

- 2 cod fillets
- 2 tablespoons olive oil
- 2 cloves garlic, minced
- 1 tablespoon chopped fresh thyme
- 1 tablespoon chopped fresh rosemary
- Salt and pepper to taste
- Lemon wedges for serving

Procedure:

1. Preheat the oven to 400°F (200°C).
2. In a small bowl, mix olive oil, minced garlic, chopped fresh thyme, chopped fresh rosemary, salt, and pepper.
3. Place the cod fillets in a baking dish and drizzle the herb mixture over them.
4. Bake in the preheated oven for about 12-15 minutes or until the cod is cooked through and flakes easily with a fork.
5. Serve the baked cod with herb crust and lemon wedges.

Grilled Lemon Garlic Shrimp

Ingredients:

- 1 pound large shrimp, peeled and deveined
- 2 tablespoons olive oil
- 2 tablespoons lemon juice
- 2 cloves garlic, minced
- 1 teaspoon lemon zest

- Salt and pepper to taste

Procedure:

1. In a bowl, toss the peeled and deveined shrimp with olive oil, lemon juice, minced garlic, lemon zest, salt, and pepper.
2. Medium-high heat should be used to preheat a grill or grill pan.
3. Grill the shrimp for about 2-3 minutes on each side or until they are opaque and cooked through.
4. Serve the grilled lemon garlic shrimp hot.

Seared Scallops with Fresh Herbs

Ingredients:

- 1 pound sea scallops
- 2 tablespoons olive oil
- 2 tablespoons chopped fresh parsley
- 1 tablespoon chopped fresh chives
- 1 tablespoon chopped fresh tarragon
- Salt and pepper to taste
- Lemon wedges for serving

Procedure:

1. With paper towels, pat the sea scallops dry before seasoning with salt and pepper.
2. In a skillet, heat olive oil over medium-high heat.
3. Add the scallops to the skillet and sear for about 2-3 minutes on each side or until they are golden brown and cooked through.
4. Remove the scallops from the skillet and toss them with chopped fresh parsley, chopped fresh chives, chopped fresh tarragon, salt, and pepper.
5. Serve the seared scallops with fresh herbs and lemon wedges.

Ingredients:

- 2 halibut fillets
- 2 tablespoons olive oil
- 1 tablespoon lime juice
- 1 teaspoon ground cumin
- 1/2 teaspoon chili powder
- Salt and pepper to taste

For the Mango Salsa:

- 1 ripe mango, diced
- 1/4 cup diced red bell pepper
- 1/4 cup diced red onions
- 2 tablespoons chopped fresh cilantro
- 1 tablespoon lime juice
- Salt and pepper to taste

Procedure:

1. In a bowl, mix olive oil, lime juice, ground cumin, chili powder, salt, and pepper to make the marinade for the halibut.
2. Place the halibut fillets in a shallow dish and coat them with the marinade.
3. The heat should be set to high before using a grill or grill pan.
4. Grill the halibut fillets for about 3-4 minutes on each side or until they are cooked through and flake easily with a fork.
5. In a separate bowl, combine diced mango, diced red bell pepper, diced red onions, chopped fresh cilantro, lime juice, salt, and pepper to make the mango salsa.

6. On top of the grilled halibut, place a large spoonful of mango salsa.

Lemon Dill Shrimp Scampi

Ingredients:

- 1 pound large shrimp, peeled and deveined
- 2 tablespoons olive oil
- 2 tablespoons lemon juice
- 2 cloves garlic, minced
- 1 tablespoon chopped fresh dill
- Salt and pepper to taste

Procedure:

1. In a bowl, toss the peeled and deveined shrimp with olive oil, lemon juice, minced garlic, chopped fresh dill, salt, and pepper.
2. Preheat a skillet over medium heat.
3. Add the shrimp to the skillet and sauté for about 2-3 minutes on each side or until they are opaque and cooked through.
4. Serve the lemon dill shrimp scampi hot.

Grilled Swordfish with Herb Butter

Ingredients:

- 2 swordfish steaks
- 2 tablespoons olive oil
- 2 tablespoons lemon juice
- 2 cloves garlic, minced
- 1 tablespoon chopped fresh thyme
- 1 tablespoon chopped fresh rosemary
- Salt and pepper to taste

For the Herb Butter:

- 2 tablespoons unsalted butter, softened
- 1 tablespoon chopped fresh parsley
- 1 tablespoon chopped fresh chives
- 1 tablespoon chopped fresh tarragon
- Salt and pepper to taste

Procedure:

1. In a bowl, mix olive oil, lemon juice, minced garlic, chopped fresh thyme, chopped fresh rosemary, salt, and pepper to make the marinade for the swordfish.
2. Place the swordfish steaks in a shallow dish and coat them with the marinade.
3. Grill or grill pan should be preheated at medium-high heat.
4. Grill the swordfish steaks for about 4-5 minutes on each side or until they are cooked through.
5. In a separate bowl, combine softened unsalted butter, chopped fresh parsley, chopped fresh chives, chopped fresh tarragon, salt, and pepper to make the herb butter.
6. Serve the grilled swordfish steaks with a dollop of herb butter on top.

Pan-Seared Tuna with Sesame Soy Glaze

Ingredients:

- 2 tuna steaks
- 2 tablespoons low-sodium soy sauce
- 1 tablespoon rice vinegar
- 1 tablespoon honey or maple syrup
- 1 tablespoon toasted sesame seeds
- 1 tablespoon sesame oil

- Salt and pepper to taste

Procedure:

1. Pat the tuna steaks dry with paper towels and season with salt and pepper.
2. Sesame oil is heated over medium-high heat in a skillet.
3. Add the tuna steaks to the skillet and sear for about 2-3 minutes on each side or until they are cooked to your desired level of doneness.
4. In a small bowl, whisk together low-sodium soy sauce, rice vinegar, honey or maple syrup, and toasted sesame seeds to make the sesame soy glaze.
5. Drizzle the glaze over the pan-seared tuna steaks.
6. Serve the pan-seared tuna with sesame soy glaze hot.

CHAPTER 10: DESERT RECIPES

Baked Apples with Cinnamon

Ingredients:

- 4 medium-sized apples (such as Granny Smith or Honeycrisp)
- 2 tablespoons honey or maple syrup
- 1 teaspoon ground cinnamon
- 1/4 cup chopped walnuts (optional)

Procedure:

1. Preheat the oven to 375°F (190°C).
2. The apples should be cored and put in a baking dish.
3. Over the apples, drizzle some honey or maple syrup.
4. Sprinkle ground cinnamon over the apples.
5. If desired, stuff the center of each apple with chopped walnuts.
6. Bake in the preheated oven for about 20-25 minutes or until the apples are tender.
7. Serve the baked apples with cinnamon warm.

Banana Oat Cookies

Ingredients:

- 2 ripe bananas, mashed
- 1 cup rolled oats
- 1/4 cup chopped nuts (such as almonds or walnuts)
- 1/4 cup dark chocolate chips (optional)
- 1/2 teaspoon ground cinnamon
- 1/4 teaspoon vanilla extract

Procedure:

1. A baking sheet should be lined with parchment paper and the oven should be preheated to 350°F (175°C).
2. In a bowl, combine mashed bananas, rolled oats, chopped nuts, dark chocolate chips (if using), ground cinnamon, and vanilla extract.
3. Mix each component in the mixture thoroughly until uniform.
4. Using a spoon, drop small portions of the mixture onto the prepared baking sheet to form cookies.
5. With the back of the spoon, slightly press each biscuit.
6. The cookies should bake for 12 to 15 minutes, or until golden brown, in the preheated oven.
7. Before serving, let the cookies cool fully on a wire rack.

Chia Seed Pudding

Ingredients:

- 1/4 cup chia seeds
- 1 cup unsweetened almond milk or coconut milk
- 1 tablespoon honey or maple syrup
- 1/2 teaspoon vanilla extract
- Fresh berries for topping

Procedure:

1. In a bowl, combine chia seeds, unsweetened almond milk or coconut milk, honey or maple syrup, and vanilla extract.
2. Stir thoroughly to distribute the chia seeds evenly.
3. Cover the bowl and refrigerate the mixture for at least 2-3 hours or overnight to allow it to thicken.
4. Stir the chia seed pudding before serving and top with fresh berries.

Baked Pears with Honey and Cinnamon

Ingredients:

- 4 ripe pears (such as Bosc or Anjou)
- 2 tablespoons honey
- 1/2 teaspoon ground cinnamon
- 1/4 cup chopped almonds or walnuts (optional)

Procedure:

1. Preheat the oven to 375°F (190°C).
2. Pears should be cut in half, with the core and seeds removed.
3. Place the pear halves in a baking dish, cut-side up.
4. Drizzle honey over the pear halves.
5. Sprinkle ground cinnamon over the pears.
6. If desired, sprinkle chopped almonds or walnuts over the pears.
7. Bake in the preheated oven for about 20-25 minutes or until the pears are tender.
8. Serve the baked pears with honey and cinnamon warm.

Almond Butter Rice Cakes

Ingredients:

- Rice cakes (gluten-free, if preferred)
- Almond butter (unsweetened and no added salt)
- Sliced bananas or berries for topping

Procedure:

1. Spread a thin layer of almond butter on each rice cake.
2. Top the almond butter rice cakes with sliced bananas or berries.
3. Serve the almond butter rice cakes as a sweet and crunchy dessert option.

Yogurt Parfait with Berries

Ingredients:

- 1 cup plain Greek yogurt (non-fat or low-fat)
- 1/2 cup mixed berries (such as blueberries, strawberries, and raspberries)
- 2 tablespoons honey or maple syrup
- 2 tablespoons granola (gluten-free, if preferred)

Procedure:

1. In a glass or dessert bowl, layer plain Greek yogurt, mixed berries, honey or maple syrup, and granola.
2. Repeat the layers if desired.
3. Serve the yogurt parfait with berries chilled.

Mango Sorbet

Ingredients:

- 2 ripe mangoes, peeled and chopped
- 1 tablespoon honey or maple syrup
- 1 tablespoon lime juice
- Fresh mint leaves for garnish (optional)

Procedure:

1. In a blender or food processor, puree the chopped mangoes, honey or maple syrup, and lime juice until smooth.
2. Mango puree should be poured into a shallow dish and frozen for at least two to three hours, or until it is hard.

3. Before serving, let the mango sorbet sit at room temperature for a few minutes to soften slightly.

4. Garnish the mango sorbet with fresh mint leaves if desired.

Coconut and Berry Chia Pudding

Ingredients:

- 1/4 cup chia seeds

- 1 cup unsweetened coconut milk

- 1 tablespoon honey or maple syrup

- 1/2 teaspoon vanilla extract

- 1/2 cup mixed berries (such as blueberries, strawberries, and raspberries)

- Unsweetened shredded coconut for topping

Procedure:

1. In a bowl, combine chia seeds, unsweetened coconut milk, honey or maple syrup, and vanilla extract.

2. Stir thoroughly to distribute the chia seeds evenly.

3. Cover the bowl and refrigerate the mixture for at least 2-3 hours or overnight to allow it to thicken.

4. Before serving, layer the chia pudding with mixed berries in individual glasses or bowls.

5. Top the chia pudding with unsweetened shredded coconut.

Dark Chocolate Dipped Strawberries

Ingredients:

- Fresh strawberries
- Dark chocolate chips (unsweetened and no added sugar)
- Chopped nuts (such as almonds or walnuts) for topping (optional)

Procedure:

1. In a microwave-safe bowl, melt the dark chocolate chips in the microwave, stirring every 30 seconds until smooth.
2. Dip each strawberry into the melted dark chocolate, coating about half of the strawberry.
3. If desired, immediately sprinkle chopped nuts over the chocolate-dipped part of the strawberry.
4. Place the chocolate-dipped strawberries on a parchment-lined tray and let them cool and set in the refrigerator for a few minutes before serving.

Baked Peaches with Greek Yogurt and Honey

Ingredients:

- 4 ripe peaches, halved and pitted
- 1 cup plain Greek yogurt (non-fat or low-fat)
- 2 tablespoons honey
- 1/4 cup chopped almonds or walnuts (optional)

Procedure:

1. Preheat the oven to 375°F (190°C).
2. Place the peach halves in a baking dish, cut-side up.
3. Bake in the preheated oven for about 15-20 minutes or until the peaches are tender.

4. Allow the baked peaches to cool slightly.

5. Fill the center of each baked peach half with a dollop of plain Greek yogurt.

6. Drizzle honey over the Greek yogurt.

7. If desired, sprinkle chopped almonds or walnuts over the yogurt and honey.

8. Serve the baked peaches with Greek yogurt and honey warm.

MEAL PLAN

DAYS	BREAKFAST	LUNCH	DINNER
1	Chia Seed Pudding with Fresh Berries	Tuna and White Bean Salad	Baked Lemon Herb Salmon with Steamed Asparagus
2	Banana Oat Cookies	Grilled Chicken and Vegetable Salad	Grilled Shrimp Skewers with Quinoa and Broccoli
3	Greek Yogurt Parfait with Berries	Tomato Basil Soup (ACID REFLUX-FRIENDLY TOMATO SOUP RECIPE)	Baked Cod with Herbs and Sautéed Spinach
4	Almond Butter Rice Cakes with Sliced Apples	Chickpea and Cucumber Salad	Lemon Dill Shrimp Scampi with Cauliflower Rice
5	Baked Apples with Cinnamon	Grilled Chicken Wrap with Hummus and Mixed Greens	Seared Scallops with Fresh Herbs and Roasted Brussels Sprouts
6	Mango Sorbet	Mediterranean Quinoa Salad	Grilled Lemon Garlic Shrimp with Brown Rice and Zucchini
7	Almond Butter and Banana Smoothie	Tuna Salad Lettuce Wraps	Baked Pears with Honey and Cinnamon and a side of Greek Yogurt
8	Greek Yogurt with Honey and Walnuts	Hummus and Veggie Wrap	Grilled Halibut with Mango Salsa and Quinoa
9	Dark Chocolate-Dipped Strawberries	Lentil and Vegetable Soup	Baked Peaches with Greek Yogurt and Honey and a side of Mixed Greens

10	Chia Seed Pudding with Mixed Berries	Grilled Vegetable and Quinoa Salad	Baked Lemon Herb Salmon with Sautéed Spinach
11	Banana Oat Cookies	Chickpea and Cucumber Salad	Grilled Chicken and Vegetable Skewers with Brown Rice
12	Greek Yogurt Parfait with Berries	Tomato Basil Soup	Seared Scallops with Fresh Herbs and Roasted Brussels Sprouts
13	Almond Butter Rice Cakes with Sliced Apples	Mediterranean Quinoa Salad	Grilled Lemon Garlic Shrimp with Cauliflower Rice
14	Mango Sorbet	Tuna Salad Lettuce Wraps	Baked Cod with Herbs and Steamed Asparagus
15	Greek Yogurt with Honey and Walnuts	Grilled Chicken Wrap with Hummus and Mixed Greens	Baked Pears with Honey and Cinnamon and a side of Greek Yogurt
16	Dark Chocolate-Dipped Strawberries	Lentil and Vegetable Soup	Grilled Halibut with Mango Salsa and Quinoa
17	Chia Seed Pudding with Mixed Berries	Grilled Vegetable and Quinoa Salad	Lemon Dill Shrimp Scampi with Brown Rice and Zucchini
18	Almond Butter and Banana Smoothie	Hummus and Veggie Wrap	Baked Lemon Herb Salmon with Sautéed Spinach
19	Baked Apples with Cinnamon	Grilled Chicken and Vegetable Salad	Grilled Shrimp Skewers with Quinoa and Broccoli
20	Banana Oat Cookies	Tomato Basil Soup	Baked Cod with Herbs and Roasted Brussels

			Sprouts

CONCLUSION

As we reach the final pages of "Reclaiming Comfort: A Journey to Freedom from Acid Reflux," it's my hope that you've found a treasure trove of solutions to overcome the challenges of acid reflux. Through the information shared in these chapters, we've discovered that an acid reflux-friendly diet isn't just a collection of recipes; it's a gateway to a life unburdened by discomfort and limitations. Remember, this journey doesn't end here. Armed with the knowledge you've gained, you now have the power to take charge of your own well-being. It's not just about the food you consume; it's about the mindful choices you make, the lifestyle adjustments you embrace, and the self-compassion you shower upon yourself.

As you embark on this path to freedom, keep in mind the small victories along the way. The first time you enjoy a flavorful meal without a hint of acid reflux, the moments when you confidently navigate food choices, and the newfound energy that propels you forward - these are all milestones on your journey. Stay curious and continue exploring the vast world of flavors that align with your well-being. Discover new ingredients, experiment with innovative recipes, and share the joy of your culinary adventures with loved ones. This isn't just about managing a condition; it's about living a life that resonates with vitality and joy.

Lastly, I'd like to express my gratitude for allowing me to be a part of your quest for freedom from acid reflux. Your commitment to prioritizing your health and well-being is inspiring, and I'm confident that you'll find the balance and comfort you deserve. So, as you turn the final page, remember that this isn't an ending; it's a new beginning. Embrace the flavors of life, nourish your body and soul, and savor the gift of a life liberated from the shackles of acid reflux.

Thank you for choosing this book. May your days be filled with vitality, and may your journey be as fulfilling as the vibrant, flavorful recipes within these pages. Wishing you a future filled with comfort, joy, and boundless possibilities. Your journey continues, and the path is yours to navigate. Bon appétit!

www.ingramcontent.com/pod-product-compliance
Lightning Source LLC
Chambersburg PA
CBHW080727260726
48660CB00010B/3724